I0765837

J. Pelegrin

80's Are The New 50's

(If you prepare in advance)

OM Publishing n.y.c.

J. Pelegrin

80's Are The New 50's

(If you prepare in advance)

Living my 80's,
Looking and Feeling like 50's

The Brain as the body
Commander in Chief

My Doctor suggested me:
People would like to read your experience

No regrets, no complaints.
Just a Happy Life!

80's Are The New 50's

(If you prepare in advance)

by J. Pelegrin

80's Are The New 50's

(If you prepare in advance)

by J. Pelegrin

TABLE OF CONTENTS

Important message to readers:

The author welcomes and encourages any comments on this book.

If you are a Amazon Premium member, you could leave your feedback on the book's page:

If you are not an Amazon Premium member, please send an email to mayavadi@aol.com with your comment.

Your words are important for new readers, to take advantage of this experience.

Thank you, very much for your cooperation and for reading it.

J. Pelegrin

About the Author: (Summary)

J. Pelegrin is a Writer, Musician, Composer, Music Producer, Filmmaker, Philosopher and God believer, although he does not practice any religion.

He lives in New York City since 1974, but before he had a successful career in the Music Business with his group "Los 4 Brillantes", with over one hundred hit records in Latin America.

In New York, he produced five hit records on the Parade scored several arrangements and played in several successful productions.

After the Music Business collapse, Jorge dedicated his full time to writing, having published three books: SAVING AMERICA THE BEAUTIFUL,

Postmodern LIBERALISM, and a novel: DEATH IS ONLY AN ILLUSION.

He also wrote a Musical Film script, and the music, for a Broadway Play officially selected at the "2015 Beverly Hills Film Festival."

His latest super-exciting Science Fiction Novel: DEATH IS ONLY AN ILLUSION is selling now at Amazon.com.

On the work: "KEEPING AMERICA GREAT!" (Revision 2) (An Evil Plan To Destroy The U.S.A. As It Is) he is leaving a testimony but overall a warning for the times ahead: We, as a Nation, must not forget how we achieved success. Although "the only permanent in life are changes," equilibrium must be kept to continue the victorious path.

J. Pelegrin

80's Are The New 50's

(If you prepare in advance)

PROLOGUE (Introduction)

Regarding health, things are more complicated than most people think.

Many issues play roles on the subject. Lifestyle, place of residence, economic situation, goals, but overall, the individual's genes, inherited from his/her family.

It is quite tricky to pinpoint strict directions on what to do or how to do it because there are so many options and desired goals as there are people. It is an individual option for sure.

However, I believe it could be interesting here, to write about the main issues as well as the peripherals which involve education, particular studies, experiences, background, lifestyles, and many other aspects that connect to the daily practice of eating and taking care of the body, like hygiene, personal care, sleeping habit, exercising and others.

Among the most important and I must be a little personal here, I am a professional musician and a writer, which as scientists, scholars and general people say, there are privileged activities, although not many of my colleagues take advantage of it. It is widely known that in the past, excesses on drugs, alcohol and a lack of care for personal care, have ruined many great artists careers, driving some of them to premature death in the worse possible conditions. But, let's lament the loss of the ones who took the wrong way, for whatever the reason and focus on the positive aspects.

It is a common thought among young artists that a considerable portion of them might prefer a short and intense life rather than a long one, where the decay of the physical body is painful to daily watch in the mirror. However, not only the artistic community is thinking and acting that way, but also, the rest of the youth has a tendency to follow the trend.

There is a fine art to age with dignity and taking advantage of the accumulated knowledge and experience of a lifetime. It is possible, and trust me, quite enjoyable. But it requires a bit of detachment from one's ego, especially assuming that the same as life, the physical body is in a constant change, where changes are the only constant. Of course, those changes are tricky, because as the body shows decaying every day, the body and mind show the fantastic experience of the knowledge acquired over the years.

Good health is the most desired status that practically all humans want to enjoy during their life.

There are a several billion dollar industries in the market selling all kinds of products, teachings, props, and tricks competing for the customer's attention and their hard-earned dollars and the choice of the good ones is as tricky as getting the desired results.

The most critical issues, apart from having good genes, as a positive start, are the eating habits and exercising. But these subjects derive from one most crucial beginning: the brain, the mind, and the desire, a product of both that will define the route to follow.

You ought to desire something for it to happen. However, it is not that simple. Many times we fight our desire instinctively, even when we know we should not do it. I guess that's why we are humans, and why we are not perfect. I am just mentioning this, but let's keep focusing on the positive.

So, a plan is necessary considering the basics. Where are we coming from, the place we live, our work or study, occupation, marital status, family, friends, and so many subjects that define our life.

I hope we are getting a clear understanding that the answers are not easy and the requirement of our will power is a must. We should strongly desire to be healthy and be ready to do the necessary things to achieve success.

I wish I could be helpful to you and deliver the proper examples and guidance to achieve this difficult task. But, remember; the success is entirely up to you!

J. Pelegrin

80's Are The New 50's

(If you prepare in advance)

CHAPTER 1

The power of the brain.

I never thought I was going to live to be over eighty years old. However, here I am, enjoying life to the fullest and healthy enough to not even think about death, at least for now.

Under the premise that our brain is the operation center of our material life, we must assume everything we think, do, feel, and planning have the roots in it. Our brain is the "think tank," and the kitchen where we cook or handle everything material. The outcome is the desire to do things.

It will be handy to clarify that our existence has two distinct parts: the material and the spiritual, although people have a misunderstanding. For instance, the brain, and its first product: the mind is material, despite some people believe they are spiritual. Well, they share one crucial issue: Consciousness, which is the nexus between the spirit soul and the physical body.

Health then is a feature of the body that commands every aspect of our behavior, considering that our actions are the communicator with other people and the evaluation tool that conforms our personality.

It is not my intention to get entangled in an argument about the separation of powers within ourselves, but at least to have a clear understanding of reality.

Of course, the mind defines everything before it becomes a desire. Although the action sometimes stays inside ourselves and other times interacts with people, the

24

decisions we make, affect our behavior and often, other people's behavior.

That is why the expression of our desires ought to be selected to separate our inner inclinations and the ones that could affect others.

This process leads the mind, and it helps to build an attitude that will support the body's health, which, of course, includes the brain, that powerful engine that keeps our bodies running.

Any changes in mood, attitude, or desire will influence our health and will generate karma reactions. Any negative thought, action or even the thought of either, will change our mood and help to define the steps that will lead us to send messages to our organs which at the same time will operate changes in their function. We could easily explain the process as a binary system of positive and negative signals that shape the permanent status of body health.

How many times our mood dictates corporal behaviors like a headache, a digestive disorder, or mental unrest? Also, muscular aches generated by bad postures or excessive usage (abuse.) Some bad news can ruin, sometimes, our digestion, even create acidity in our stomach.

A few days ago, in a visit to one of my dear doctors, after a comment about my body's general good condition, he asked me? Why don't you write a book about it? I think many people could use your feedback!

My first reaction was: why anybody would read my book, being that I am not a famous writer and a little far away from the days of my music success? So, the initial rejection became a consideration, and a few days later, I decided at least, to initiate writing an "essay," to see how would it read.

It is true, my health and my looks are superb, despite my three strokes, which I had a full recovery from them and my scoliosis, which Dr. Steven G. Halley and his team helps me to manage.

When meeting new people sometimes, just for kicks, I ask how old do they think I am, most responses, if they don't have a clue that leads them to an educated guess, like some references to documents or past

26

experiences is more or less the same: Oh, you might be about 54 or 55 years old, a flattering answer which after it, I reveal my real age. I also keep all my hair, although white since my twenties, which is part of my good genes.   I consider lightly dishonest to cheat on the age, and besides, it is much better people being surprised about the state of my body than thinking you are a "common age cheater." The fact is that age as a few years ago walking with a friend ten years younger than me; we commented:

"Age is just a number." And I added: we will defeat it. My friend, a professional dancer, is keeping teaching dance classes almost daily, after receiving a hip replacement on both sides. It is a matter of attitude and will power.

My beloved Spiritual Master, Bhaktivedanta Swami Prabhupada used to joke: My dear disciples, every morning as you wake up, we should grab an old shoe and beat

our heads a few times. That will help us to listen to our brain and keep our minds focused on our duty. Of course, to maintain our body is an essential one. God, or Krishna, as I like to call him <it is said in the Vedas, that we are in charge of our body and its maintenance is an everyday duty we must religiously engage.>

When my dear mother was in a hospital bed, after a stroke and still unconscious, examining her body, me and my wife at the time, she commented that at 83 years old, her skin, particularly her feet, were in great shape. Then, I remembered that she used to encourage me to

"think of your feet," at every moment. Move them and exercise them to keep the blood flowing. "if you forget them, they won't like it and quickly decay.'

It is common to see older people suffering and even dealing with deformations due to a lack of proper care. I often massage my feet and even wearing shoes; I keep moving them to avoid inflammation or numbness. Also, we must continuously exercise our hands and fingers. As a musician who plays the keyboards an at present daily use a typewriter or computer board, I have routinely been exercising my fingers all my life. That is one of the many advantages of being a musician. The notion that musicians live longer and enjoy a better life is something we daily hear thru the grapevine. I could not agree more about it. I vigorously defend such a thesis.

Music is a product of mathematics. Algorithms define the complex phrasing and elaborated sound vibrations that for centuries, we were only able to feel without a graphic explanation, other than the notes on a staff, designed by the genius of Pythagoras. Digital music has expanded the frontiers allowing us to be able to 'see' music in addition to hear it. We are living an age of exciting opportunities that continue to develop our minds in different dimensions. Unfortunately, "some mind Corsairs" are trying to spoil the daydream by stretching the safe zones looking for dangerous ways that inevitably will defeat the experimental purposes in many ways.

Science is theorizing with at least ten dimensions, as explained in the study of 'String Theory.' It is considered necessary to understand the multi-universes system or 'multiverse,' recently discovered by scientists.

However, without any scientific nowadays are recklessly engaging considerations, many groups in purely speculative experiments much too controversial for most people, especially Conservatives. Perhaps the word "Conservative" is misunderstood because it is not a matter of staying glued to the past, but over that base, opening to a sensitive exploration of new avenues without losing the main route drawn by our creator to cross the ocean of life and reaching the other side of the shore, to another world, in a different dimension. A spiritual existence, of course, I don't expect the readers to accept my philosophy, although I strongly suggest taking an in-depth look at it. It worked for me. Here is a quotation which I ignore the source. However, it is real and somehow identifies a reality: "Life is not a journey to the grave to arrive safely in a pretty and well-preserved body, but rather to skid in broadside -- thoroughly used up, totally worn out, and loudly proclaiming:.. <Wow! What a ride!>"

Certainly, the ride is better when one is healthy! Therefore, to achieve such a goal, it is necessary to follow a discipline of essential body maintenance.

In the morning, while I am showering, applying safe hot water to my lower back, I thank God for a whole day without pain. The intense hot-water on my lower back is like a body tune-up, to continue the journey in the best possible condition. Although it is better not taking pain medicines, sometimes I do take 100 mg. of Diclofenac Sodium, a non-addictive muscle relaxant, after some physical strength. Then, some moisturizing

cream to my feet and lower legs, and ready to go!

Being born in Uruguay, South America has had its pros and cons.

On the positive side, besides the enormous advantage of having amazing parents and lovable relatives, life in this tiny but great country was excellent. Then, the Left ruined it, after the Right-wing politicians abused their functions and practically invited Socialism and Communism to convince the Uruguayan people to try another different governing system. Uruguay was an Oasis in the middle of a vast undeveloped South American sub-Continent that the rest of the World used to call 'the Switzerland of America.' Let's remember that America is a Continent and the United States of America has adopted a short of defining its name as "America," which for many other Americans seems to be a bit confiscating or aggressive appropriation.

Today, Uruguay is a shadow of the past, to sad to comment about it. It is no longer the 'Switzerland of America,' thanks to the changes by the Left. I grew up under the thought that everything in moderation was the safe way to go on thru my existence, although my compatriots' example differed. Uruguay was known at the time, to have among the best red meat in the World and it was the main staple and daily meal for the whole country. Red meat consumption was creating an abnormally high colon cancer disease and deprived the body to have a balanced nutritious meal as conscious people, and scientists recommend.

There were times of ignorance

mainly carried by uneducated immigrants escaping European

wars and consequential poverty. So, that was the reality. However,

some people, educated enough, became politicians, at the beginning of the twenties century, showing a sincere dedication to maintaining a decent country. They were eager to succeed and enjoying life within the limitations set by its small size, the type of immigrants coming to the land, adding to the remains of the descendants from the Spanish 'Conquistadores' that stayed on the ground.

There was a peaceful bunch of simple people, guided by some well-educated leaders with good intentions, at least in the beginning. Then, perhaps because of an abundance of food (cows meat), natural to produce without any efforts, spoiled the newer generations and corruption exploded ending with what it was initially a beautiful country's experience.

However, there were some positive experiences in my early life that helped me to improve my knowledge and self-development.

The forties and fifties were plenty of good things happening in my life, overall with primary human education, socially correct, a loving family, some good friends and a prosperous country selling its primary production, cows meat, excessively valued in a World hit by wars. Due to the Worldwide armed conflicts in Europe and the East, their destroyed prairies by the war and the cattle disappeared together with the farms, also unable to grow vegetables and fruits creating hunger among locals having to import meat to survive. So, Uruguay became wealthy as the producer of the best quality red meat in the World. That caused a temporary bonanza in the economy, at present, long gone.

So, my youth was very good, indeed, and before the regression started, I left the country, looking to develop my artistic skills, with an objective set in one country: The United States of America.

However, a successful career as a musician-composer-arranger-producer delayed my preset goal for a few years and previous to a few short trips to the South of the USA, I finally arrived in New York City in 1974.

My relationship with the most magnificent city in the World was love at first site. Coming from a small Capital, Montevideo, Uruguay, it was not a shock being in NYC, and immediately, I found similarities that made my life easier, despite my lack of English Language skills. However, with the help of a dictionary and watching the memorable Johnny Carson, with his impeccable English diction and vocabulary, I learned the language in one year. Somebody had told me: If you learn 300 words in English, you will be able to have a conversation with any local people. And it is true. Of course, it is not the goal, but it is a starter. Especially that in 1974, not many people in the city could speak Spanish or even understand it.

Luckily, within three months of adjusting to the City life, I got an opportunity to record at CBS Columbia Records International and to be sponsored by its President, Walter Yetnicoff, an icon in the industry.

Unfortunately, with the recording in process, Columbia Records CEO died, and Yetnicoff promoted to CEO. Shortly, I received a call from him communicating the news and also advising me that I had to shift my dependence to another Executive coming from the UK, which didn't like my project: a combination of Latin Music and Funk. However, I managed to get out of my contract and find the singers to my production in a thriving group.

The recording was a hit; my first music success in the USA, a short five months after my arrival. Not bad.

Before traveling to New York, and while enjoying seven continuous years of success, traveling to more than 150 cities and Towns in Mexico, I became a vegetarian. First, I stopped eating red meat, a few months later I gave up chicken and fish, although I continued to eat eggs. a year then I was a total dairy/vegetarian, meaning refraining from all meats and having dairy products as a primary source of protein.

New York helped me to be a dairy-vegetarian. Fruits and vegetables of the best quality were widely available at the time, helping to continue my diet.

Before I began my vegetarianism, I had severe problems with sinusitis, common-colds, stomach disarrays, and also liver issues. As the new diet progressed, my body responded, and all the mentioned problems disappeared with time. Nowadays, the last time I remember having the flu is seven years ago, when doctors convinced me to get a "flu shot." I had a severe flu issue that lasted three months, in the summertime. Of course, I never retook the vaccine. As of today, I still haven't have the flu or a common cold.

Excess of mucus is a common cause of infection in the rest of your body, that starts on your throat and travels down into the stomach and other organs.

Watching what you eat helps to avoid its excess. Although the body needs some mucus, too much can cause severe damage.

80's Are The New 50's

(If you prepare in advance)

CHAPTER 2

The big city challenge.

Life in New York City requires exercising. It is something most people agree. There are plenty of Gyms of all prices imaginable so, there are no arguments to keep a sedentary life which will inevitably drive you to overeat and gaining weight. So, I have made a kind of religious commitment to go to the gym at least four to five times a week. In the summer, I frequently replace the Gym session with a five miles walk in Central Park that is also a way to oxygenate my lungs and add some healthy nature input to my brain. Remember that the brain is the commander in chief of your body so, it also needs food, of course of different nature, and Nature is the best way to feed it.

Exercising as you age, is quite challenging to continue, and the brain quickly finds excuses to skip it or even quit the pace. However, discipline helps you to remind that you should drag your body to

the Gym under any circumstance. Once you are at it, then you get the energy to exercise that before getting there you thought you couldn't have. It is one of the rules that keep you healthy living in a big city.

Not only that but the eating habits you must acquire, especially choosing the quantities that you eat, as well as the time you do it.

Excessive quantities of food and sugary drinks are the main reasons we get fat.

Think that the body only processes and retains the number of nutrients it needs to function healthily and safely, discarding the rest. There are folks that because they think carrot juice, for instance, is beneficial to your health, especially your eyes, they overtake it. I've seen people with their skin turning "carrot color," and even leaving stains in objects they touch because of the excess of carotene.

So, since I was a child, I heard my mom, over and over telling me: "everything in moderation."

Gaining weight is very easy. You can add two or three pounds in a day or even more. Continuing with a reckless diet can drive you to add ten or fifteen pounds in a week in a breeze. However, to lose the excess gained, it might take a few weeks or months under a severe sacrifice that is controlling what you eat and savagely reducing the portions. So, remember that you can indulge yourself on occasion, but the next day you must get rid of the weight you gained. Following this simple rule will help you to enjoy the food you love, but restricting your diet on the next journey, when the excess remains in your body in the form of 'waste' but it wasn't absorbed in the form of fat yet.

If you follow this simple rule, trust me; it makes your life much more comfortable and pleasant. And it is, again, moderation.

Drinking alcohol is another easy way to gain weight. I prefer not to advise this habit because it is so personal and painful to manage that hundreds of books have been written and people continue to drink until they can't take it anymore, so, let's add my advice to the general rule of: "everything in moderation, please."

Also, smoking cigarettes is a danger to health, and lately, vaping, which at the beginning was considered safe, has been the cause of several deaths, after some people developed serious lung condition. Of course, youngsters, have been mixing the chemical sold with the vaping devices with other drugs, sold in the streets with no medical supervision or Government control.

Staying healthy is so important that we must watch any substance that enters our body, because the consequences could be lethal.

When people often say: I don't understand why I gain weight. I eat so little. O.K. you eat very little but also, you eat the wrong food. Because regardless of metabolic disruptions and other issues that cause a disturbance in people's body, honestly, and I am risking to be a little nasty with this comment. If there were a way for people to gain weight and be healthy without eating, the African or Asian countries with famine problems would give all their wealth to be able to put such a system in practice.

It is a simple ruling. If you overeat, the body will transform the unnecessary food into fat and will eliminate the rest.

It is hard for some people to understand that the body doesn't need an enormous amount of food to survive. Also, a simple fact: the body functions much better when the weight is less. Simple rules indicate that anybody carrying overweight needs much more energy than moving a lighter body. It sounds simple. However, not many people accept the validity of such a simple matter. Something called "gluttony" is the primary cause of eating disorders. Eating with the eyes is not a good idea. Select your portions accordingly with your metabolic capabilities. Keep in mind what it was already said: You can overeat on occasions, but restraint is needed the next day or two.

We should consider each body is a different universe in itself, and there are infinite types of behavior and unique forms of living.

The creator has a way to make every single body so particular and with different needs that it is impossible making an only rule of behavior.

But there is a 'common sense' which describes a set of rules that over time have been proved of utility to maintain the body healthy and in functional operation for a long time.

I must insist that the brain is the center of operations, and it issues the orders that make the right moves for a successful endeavor.

Many people resources to Yoga, to achieve the peace of mind that allows them to succeed in life. Meditation brings inner peace, stability, and those are essential components of a healthy body.

There are many types of Yoga styles that go from hard to achieve

physical exercises that help to relax the muscles to liberate the inner energy, to others that begin with breathing techniques. Others recommend sexual practices thru different positions that bring you in contact with your sexual self, as well as other schools with more intricate methods, all them looking for a sense of inner peace, relaxation in search of physical happiness. Let's remember that the mind is part of the physical body.

The body health is related to all the above, and the choices are so personal, that once again, I refrain from counseling, which is better than the other. However, there is a different kind of Yoga: "Bhakti Yoga," which is essentially a God's adoration in the body of Krishna (the preferred name of

God by Indian People.) It is a spiritual exercise that aims to elevate your consciousness to be with God at all times by prayers and offerings of flowers and food to specific deities.

There are no limits to what people use to achieve happiness. Every single one of them, in one way or the other, are involved in the process of maintaining a healthy body.

It is not a matter of how many years you can live, but the quality of life that you desire to accompany you on your journey.

I have a desire to live as far as my brain allows me to function in a way that I can enjoy being alive; no more than that. I desire that God takes me away as soon as my brain functions commence to decay.

Since I believe in life after death, I am confident that the best way to transition between the different worlds, is in a smooth change of levels within the Multiverse.

It is of course, not a matter of pure speculation since science has already confirmed the existence of thousands of universes, but besides this latest scientific discovering, the ancient Vedas, written fifty-five hundred years ago, extensively described millions of universes, containing thousands of worlds spread across the infinite that we call space. Infinite is a complex word that our brains have trouble to process because there are no measures available to size limitless or boundless settings. We must remember Albert Einstein saying that "everything is relative to the point of observation." If we move, everything changes.

The reader must think: What has this to do with health?

And yes, everything has to do with health, but mainly the attitude one has to life and our approach that position us in the point of observation.

Even if it is transitional, it will have a direct effect on our body.

I intended from the beginning when I began writing this book, not to get extremely complicated, but I find impossible, at least to me, to write just a dietary routine, because that is not an intelligent way to pass some experience to my readers.

So far, I assume that even in this Chapter, I've got a little off of a simplistic approach, I hope I didn't lose the course of sanity and good practice. I hope.

So, life in New York City operated a change in my life like no other period had before. The City has a special magnet that attracts people so intensely like no other place in the World.

People do anything to stay in New York City, to work, study, live, even the boldest attempt to raise a family. The economic issue is the critical factor and the individual's ability to generate the money needed to stay in the City, is the key element. (I mean, New York City, not the suburbs,) which I exclude not for discrimination purposes but because there is a profound difference living in the Island than residing in the Boroughs. Only after experiencing both ways, one gets to know the real contrast.

Manhattan is magic, a Disney World-like place, but real. Health is a concern; however, thousands are practically eating from the garbage containers with no health concerns, refusing Government home shelters, preferring sleeping in the subways, train stations, street alleys, Subway vents, park benches or any imaginable places, but consistently refuse to live in public shelters. The City has tried everything to tempt homeless people to sleep in Government shelters. Everything has failed. Mainly the complaints are that other folks steal from them, quarrels and they mention other personal problems. But the main difficulty nowadays is drugs, hard drugs. A severe epidemic of opioids and fentanyl is decimating the homeless like it is impossible to understand. I believe that those desperate human beings have the opposite desire to what I have, and probably most readers would have. They don't want to be healthy. They want to succumb to life, to die, and they perhaps don't dare to commit direct suicide. It is heartbreaking to realize it, but I can not find another answer. Drugs are a form of delaying death by creating a dream-like that allows them to transition without conscientious reality.

Once again, I am falling out of the simple line, but I intend to compare the parameters enclosing the health system in the different groups.

I insist that the brain is the center of the body. But we also must acknowledge the existence of an element that links the body with the spirit-soul. It is, of course, a complicated issue to digest although there is no other explanation to define it.

In my mind, the only thing that differentiates a live person with a dead one is that the living person is moving and exercising the rest of its capable functions. The dead body is soul-less, meaning that that energy that once was driving it and making possible movements, even brain functions are gone. Where? Who knows? But maybe in some place at some time, even in another dimension, could be found. Consciousness is the link between the brain in the body with the spirit soul, that unimaginable connection that unifies the whole.

50

It is fascinating just thinking about and so scary to many people that only mentioning the fact of such existence could bring chills and unrest to the unprepared.

Mental health is a current issue that even scientists have trouble to study, in my opinion, because it is not part of just the material World. It transcends the barriers of what we know and transport us to the brinks of surreality. Once again when we begin to think of the spirit world, we are entering the unknown, the mystery, with all the surprises and perilous chances that our minds could enter a street alley without an exit. Only the healthy ones with a firm concept of body care and the proper link to the spirit thru conscience may be able to handle it.

It is tough to identify who can face the challenge and who can't.

Many folks have lost it while trying, especially when the physical body is not prepared for the task. It is always handy to enjoy good health to achieve success, at least to have a grasp of reality.

Therefore, healthy life will not only show in your appearance but also will give you the ability to manage mind issues with confidence and resolve.

A healthy mind in a healthy body will complete the circle: A healthy body will keep a brain healthy, and that elevates the consciousness to the spirit level.

80's Are The New 50's

(If you prepare in advance)

CHAPTER 3

The philosophy connection.

One crucial issue has helped me to keep my sanity, my mind healthy, and also my body: Studying Philosophy; Mainly Vedic Philosophy and Vedic Science. Immersing myself in the Vedic Literature and Vedic Science has become the core of my knowledge, which includes how to handle complex issues efficiently.

"Simple living and high thinking" is the key which our Spiritual Master,

Bhaktivedanta Swami Prabhupada hammered in my brain.

Also the celebrated boys from Liverpool: The Beatles radically changed their lives after meeting such a great Soul. I could not thank enough this giant man in his fragile small body to appear in my way at the right moment. So the Beatles are also grateful to Swami Prabhupada. He taught by example, as the real Acharyas do.

He eat very little, all vegetables and fruits prepared in the Indian cuisine style. No meat, of course. Dairy products, as an essential nutritional balance component and although he loved sweets, limited the intake accordingly with good safety practices.

He didn't sleep much; only three or four hours and worked most of the journey, either studying the Sanskrit Vedic texts, translating them to the English Language or writing his books.

His main exercising was walking, but we must have present that he was not an ordinary person, with a super-intense inner life which probably shortened his physical existence. He died at 76 of kidney failure. That was his fate.

This tall man in a tiny body left an incredible legacy that only privileged people could follow 100%, but his example is golden, and we must grab whatever we can as per our ability to learn.

Meeting him and learning about his teachings was the start of a new and productive life. He changed me forever. Of course, I had to detach myself from many old habits.   His education severely diminished my ego and expanded my spirit soul and the understanding of God's Consciousness or 'Krishna Consciousness' as he liked to name it.

It is not my intention to preach religion or become a guru. I am just telling a story that changed my life, my habits, and my future. I don't pretend that you do the same as I did; however, you can take whatever could be positive for you and ignore the rest. That is part of my philosophy.

For instance, when somehow I recommend people to read the Vedic Literature, I make a sharp point. The Sanskrit Language and even the translations to the English Language that carry the original literary style in which it was written, mentioned, along with the text, an array of places, personalities, deities, fantastic setup, imaginary situations. All this, immensely complicate the understanding of its philosophy, the most crucial part of its legacy.

It is convenient to start getting to know the philosophical part of the Vedic consciousness, and then, maybe with the help of an expert, get to the details in the intricate, beautiful verses and descriptions of its magical knowledge.

It is worth it if you like deep learning. There is no other school of Literature that comes close to the Vedas. It is an in-depth education if you know how to extract its philosophical wealth.

When you acquire the know-how, then you will apply it to daily life and amazingly confirm that it works perfectly and rationally.

After meeting Srila Prabhupada, although I was already a partial vegetarian, I began studying Vedic philosophy and rearranged my life to a more orderly schedule. My mind began adjusting my goals, and my health improved accordingly with the changes. One significant improvement was applying the "portion" ruling.

I remember, a few years ago, one of my doctors remind me to watch my weight. Then, he asked me to describe my diet and the portions I was taking. Well, my favorite food is pasta in all forms and recipes, although salads are the perfect complement. So, describing my intake, I mention a quarter coin as the standard portion. He looked at me and said: "OK. Why don't you try a replacement for other elements of pasta, other than wheat? Nowadays there are plenty of products with much less carbohydrate value." I responded: I don't like replacement. I don't eat only to feed my body. Food, to me, is enjoyable, and some alternatives aren't. My doctor then said, well, then you can take, instead of a quarter of uncooked pasta, a nickel. What about that. So, that conversation made me think about changing the way I was looking at food, and since that day, I have the routine to measure the quantity of pasta I cook. Well, almost always, I must confess, sometimes I overeat, but as I said before, the next day, I try to patch-up my mistakes fasting or reducing my intake.

In sum, I manage to keep my weight decently.

Also, sugar is a sure way to gain pounds if you abuse it. Although there is an old Indian say joking that: "Sugar is not good for your body, but is very good for your Soul." Usually, I take my morning coffee, the only time I have it, without any sugar. But, Ice cream, the one with tons of sugar, is my favorite. Oops! Being a diabetic, I don't understand how is it that sugar doesn't increase my glucose levels. I also try to keep my portions to the minimum so, I can continue to indulge in this favorite dessert.

Fortunately, I am not a fan of cakes, which besides sugar, contain a real killer: carbs.

It is a delicate task that I can keep my weight in a number which allows me to be healthy and with enough energy to keep writing, making music, and living a good life.

Of course, I keep mental health and spiritual life to be the primary role of my existence.

Lately, things have become more difficult due to politics and the deep division among our neighbors. It is a shame that political differences are deeply dividing the American people. The abortion issue is also a controversial theme that it is hard to understand when in one hand, we have the fact that not enough babies are born at this time to keep our society growing. However, there is a frantic attempt to make abortions free until birth. Not only that but now some states are pushing to allow babies that failed abortion to be subject to the parents and doctors decision, to kill them. Blatant infanticide! Life is an incredible gift from our creator, and some politicians are dismissing that miracle of life, to satisfy their uncontrollable material desires, especially power.

While our economy is asking, better said, screaming that we need more people in our country because the jobs available are more than the available workers, and it seems this situation will continue in years to come. Factory jobs are returning to our country, and we need skilled workers to fill the need.

Illegal aliens, mostly primitive and unskilled males, are entering our borders without control, and that is not a good sign. I don't want to get into politics, because this book is not about it. However, I just had to mention these facts to keep it real. The state of mind created by these events are also mitigating our attitudes and actions, and therefore, our mind is sending signals to our body accordingly with the feelings emanating from it. It is complicated, I know, but it has become part of our daily life. It is horrible seeing in social media friends for life, unfriending others because of politics, couples parting ways, family members fighting, and kids are watching those behaviors, learning from these abnormal social times.

All of the above is also part of our actions and affecting our diet, our social behavior, and our health.

The present should be a time for reflection. We must clear our differences and begin to act in conjunction, retaking our old sense of country, patriotism, returning to familiar icons like our flag, which our soldiers, carry with love and devotion thru the battlefields, defending our democratic values and lifestyle.

We should send most politicians back to school, to re-learn the basics of decent living. The fight for power has been spoiled, taking a brutal way of insults, attacking rivals with lies, twisting the reality and lately, adopting anti-democratic political ideas, that our Nation fought with our youngsters lives for decades.

We must keep the initial thought of our Founding Fathers, that designed and made possible the best Nation on Earth, that for 243 years have driven us thru brave oceans, severe winters, and suffocating scolding summers, being the most desired place on Earth to reside, work, study and raise a family. Millions of illegal aliens are proof of it, having risked death crossing the Ocean in dinghy boats, paying "coyotes" to cross the border, get into jam-packed trucks with no ventilation, killing many, and other kinds of tricks. Those resulted, accordingly with some estimates, 30 million people living illegally in our country.

The USA is not perfect, but we used to aim to perfection until now, where the values have gotten mixed up, and we seem not to have a smooth exit from the actual mess.

Is that part of the confusion? The spiritual trouble that those modern "Buccaneers," I mentioned before is experimenting without any control, looking for material satisfaction, where the real place to look for it is the other part of the self: The spiritual life.

Greed, easy ways to make money, dishonesty, and 'getting away with murder,' have replaced good practices we used to prefer. Is this going to be the standard for the future? I hope not. But we better start now to change the course, or future generations are going to miss the best part of being in the United States of America. The sense of community, working for one cause, pulling together to the same side, and appreciating what God has left to us to enjoy. This Material World, its Nature, and the living entities: its inhabitants.

The related events have changed everything in our country, including living habits, our goals in life, and the teachings we are giving to children.

The peril is visible, affecting our lives on everything. Our schedule, communication with our neighbors, friends, relatives. And world, the first thing I wonder is our youngsters. What are we leaving them? What are our teachings? When we see aberration after aberration, and I cannot overlook what I saw yesterday.

Public Libraries are sponsoring Drag Queens (what should be exclusively an adult entertainment) lecturing children as young as two years old, indoctrinated on a practice that they are years away from beginning to understand?

I am not condemning homosexual practice: however, to pollute such young kids minds with sex culture? That is not in my books or any rationale sense of civilization.

While we are seeing the results of some people who have lost their north, the excess of liberty in the USA, or better said, the misuse of freedom trying to please personal deviations is ruining our culture. Maybe our Founding Fathers were a little naive and thought the old-style would prevail, and every citizen was going to work toward unity, love, country, and family with God in the center, has encountered at this time, atheists and God-haters that the only thing they have in mind is destruction. Health, once again, starts by teaching children to live a life of wellness, practicing a culture that begins with the pureness of mind, at least in the beginning. Life development itself will teach them the rest.

Although some States are trying to teach kids to eat well, especially the ones that come from low-income families, the efforts are not focusing the real world and, also, the different opinions about something that everybody has a different one.

One thing I find positive is the general concept that kids should know the values of vegetables on their diet, that sugar is not for excess consumption, and meat intake has severe consequences for the body.

However, as mentioned before, I don't want to preach any preferences, because I practice them, but I also have the right to be honest and express my opinion and how I feel about it.

This book is about what I feel and look on my eighties, and of course, my feelings are the part of the focus. Preaching is insisting and recommending something; however, exposing my preferences is only a guide that could be taken or left aside.

I firmly believe that education is the main effort to embed in children's brain. However, the options for everything available should stand available so; they can see the differences and choose the right ones, of course after the proper education is presented and making sure has been understood by kids and their parents. Otherwise, the whole endeavor could turn useless.

But remember that the power of the brain is essential to life. Philosophy is the key to learn and to understand life and the meanings and options along the way, that will drive us not only to physical wellness but also spiritual health.

As mentioned before, "A healthy mind in a healthy body" is the best choice.

80's Are The New 50's

(If you prepare in advance)

CHAPTER 4

A new diet, a new life.

Adopting my new diet wasn't easy, especially reducing the portions to almost hunger; that was the initial feeling.

When you have an eating habit, your brain sets a regular schedule, and even your stomach makes room for what is supposed to take in.

As mentioned before, the brain is the center of operations and who commands the desire, including what to eat.

It is necessary to apply a firm will power to change eating habits. Conduct is fundamental.

Modern life offers the most considerable array of foods, available at a significant inexpensive cost and even delivered at your doorsteps in New York City, and even inside your home, in suburban areas.

Also, the food display in most city stores is particularly appealing to our eyes, smell, and taste.

However, after the decision to change my eating schedule, I began to enjoy my new routine and choice of foods, as well as the new right portions, hoping that would help to maintain my body in shape, healthy and happy.

Under the understanding that the cells in our body replenish every seven days, I began to feel some changes, although not physically yet, but in feelings. If you pay attention to your brain, it issues some subtle signals, but sensible to our senses. Our brain is a fantastic piece of natural technology.

Once we process brain signals thru the mind transformed into desire, we are ready for the change, and the physical body starts adjusting to the new goal. Of course, temptations are on our way 24/7 and our commitment must prevail at all times, with some exceptions, that as explained before, is not good to accumulate. It is convenient to follow simple rules, and we must compensate our "misbehaviors," with the following day restraint, in quantity, caloric contains, carbohydrates count, or merely fasting. If you don't do that, the body will absorb the extra food as fat, and remember that getting rid of fat is not easy. It requires a more strenuous effort than merely getting rid of food in the intestine track.

You might think this is a silly way to keep a healthy weight;? It is the easiest one I know; if you follow some kind of discipline.

There are seven essential factors for a balanced diet: carbs, protein, fat, fiber, vitamins, minerals, and water.

I will avoid counseling what types of food are the best. Being a Dairy-Vegetarian, as I established before, I have personal preferences, but I leave up to the reader to choose their favorites. I would only remark that water is the most important; the avoidance of excess of fats comes second, and controlling carbs are fundamental, mainly to keep healthy glucose levels. Keep sugars intake low.

After my eating habits became a new usual way, my exercising schedule a regular, I recovered an energy level that I thought was gone for good.

I should admit that I also started taking an almost daily dose of Whey Protein, that helped me to elevate my energy levels considerably. I consume the protein powder, without abusing quantities or frequency. Periodically.

I am no fan of additional vitamin intake, although lately, by doctor's prescription, I am taking Iron and Vitamin B-12, which it seems my body always had a deficiency. I remember when I was a child, doctors often prescribing me B-12.

Then, I stopped it, and lately, thru a Lab. test, my doctor discovered I needed a supplement of it. A lack of Iron is common in people on a vegetarian diet. Animal products are the most common source of the mineral. However, you can found it in vegetables and beans. Also, taking iron pills (I take a compound coming from plants, not containing any animal product) has to be taken in conjunction with vitamin C, which helps the iron absorption into the body. The complex I consume has a dose of vitamin C among other minerals and amino acids. Besides that; I daily take a glass of orange juice in the morning.

Following the doctor's counseling has always been a regular practice, which I recommend to everyone — conducting a blood test at least every six months dramatically helps. Especially if you have Diabetes, (I test Diabetes 2, lightly) my diabetes killer is carbs, not sugar.

Salt is a necessary nutrient our body needs, although in the right quantities. Too much salt brings some problems, including heart disease, thru the hardening of our vessels. Excess of fat accumulates in the hardening veins and block the blood passage, a sure killer if unattended. However, salt is excessively demonized. Late scientific studies found out that certain types of salt, as Grey Sea Salt and other varieties, have curative properties, especially on skincare, improving dental health, relief from rheumatoid arthritis, muscle cramps, psoriasis, and osteoarthritis. It also helps in providing help from acne and rhino sinusitis, and even certain types of cancer. Furthermore, it is beneficial for exfoliation, nasal, and eyewash, and an improved electrolytic balance of the body.

It also has healing properties that play a vital role in maintaining the acid-alkali ratio, regular heartbeat, and relaxed sleep, along with providing relief from fatigue.

Of course, as my motto goes, everything in moderation. Even if beneficiary for our health, we should not abuse it.

Grey Sea Salt, which I discovered not too long ago, also has a way to improve and enhance food flavors. The only inconvenience is its natural wetness which, of course, also has a plus: it is free of additional calcium and iodine.

There are inexpensive sea salt mills, rust-free with no metal parts, to help dispense it.

Sugar is another concern. The body needs sugar in small quantities. Raw sugar, although it presents a sometimes heavy flavor, that some people dislike (I don't mind it), it is much better, healthier than white refined sugar. It might substantially change the coffee flavor if you are a caffeine lover. But, once again, everything in moderation is advised. I, personally, don't use sugar in my coffee, something that not many people may agree. I don't regularly add sugar to anything, except when I make blended fruit shakes, as Banana and Milk, or Strawberry-Banana, with crushed ice. Both delicious. I like them sweet.

Being on a dairy/vegetarian diet has helped me to avoid sinusitis, a problem I always had when I used to eat meat. I previously wrote about this inconvenience that brings an excess of mucose to the body.

In general, foods that are too acid are not very healthy. A well-balanced intake is always advisable.

Spices are an old-fashioned way to help a healthy body and even in some cases, to improve the status. There is an essential part of the ancient Ayurveda Medicine, thousands of years old healing practice in India, and around the World based on spices and herbs that we generally use for cooking. For instance, it is well known that Turmeric, Cayenne pepper, Ginger, Cinnamon, Cloves, Sage, and Rosemary, are useful anti-inflammatory aids.

Turmeric, Ginger, and Cardamon are outstanding help as antibiotics.

I could go on, although the reader can have better information on Google, thru dedicated pages or dozens of books published with ample technical details. It is my intention only to raise awareness on the subject.

We must keep in mind the primary goal of my message:

Helping my readers to have a better life, especially aging in style, gradually adding physical activity with mental, and spiritual, thru a consciousness connection. If you try it, you will see, it works.

I must emphasize to use your brain and follow the natural wisdom that will help you to achieve your daily goals.
Listening and following to your doctor's instructions and counseling is smart and always advisable. Scheduling a doctor's visit every six months is an assurance that you are cutting eventualities to a minimum. Health is not a game anymore. It is undoubtedly not something left only to destiny or fate. Nowadays, science has come an extraordinarily long way and made prevention of many illnesses real and at hand for most individuals concerned with it.
Exercising is no longer a fashion activity. It is a total necessity, especially if you live in a City. I remind you the pop say: "If you don't use it, you lose it."

Some men, even at a young age give-up sports or training vigorously, choosing a 'six-pack,' heavy liquor, smoking and eating recklessly. They grow a big belly and lose the appeal to women, and themselves when they look in the mirror, causing psychological damage to negatively affecting their whole life.

Women, also follow the same path, although in a lesser quantity, since they are more inclined to 'Look good,' especially as they age. Ignorance of facts and especially failure finding the will power within themselves are frequent. Learning what I've been writing about the brain being the commander in chief inside the body, is a life-changing factor, reserved to privileged people who refuse to take the skid road, and decide to curb their appetite, drug abuse, alcohol consumption in excess or even becoming a "couch potato.'

In recent past times, keeping the younger looks was seen as a vanity, and especially married men wouldn't pay attention.

Marriages were seen as a taken for granted social "contract," and looks were considered superficial, unimportant or banal.

However, since the T.V. age progressed and the Internet helped to create Social Media, the image became more important, changing lifestyles, communication between people, and even isolating them in a self-made cocoon where dialogue got shorten and superficial. False identities began cheating and misleading, causing old friends to get more distant and in some cases

ending longtime relationships due

to political differences. Unfortunately, these are the signs of modern life.

However, there is a positive side of it, bringing some people together, ending some fellows isolation and entertainment to older folks.

People, conscious that looks were becoming more important, began to see that being in shape was a necessary tool for those rare cases of communication, gyms sprouted out all over the country, and a general need to get in good, healthy condition became more desired.

So, the new Millennium brought some radical changes to our culture. Looking at the positive ones, the tremendous advancement in science and technology, are operating a dramatic transition, that it seems endless and complicated to keep track of it. Among them, cyber tech, communications, space science, and an increasing acceptance of Philosophy by the scientific community, are the most outstanding.

Just a few years ago, Spiritual issues were rejected as Philosophy, in a derogatory way, considering them lesser than scientific and unrelated to facts. However, as old forgotten scriptures proved to carry in-depth knowledge, and many events narrated in the ancient documents confirmed an actual link to scientific experiments performed by modern science, gradually, the advanced scientists commenced studying some of the old texts. Especially the Vedas, adopting specific theories and inserting them into new investigations, that in some cases drove them into surprising discovering.

I am not about giving a lecture about science; nevertheless, as I wrote before, I intend to bring awareness about issues that I have learned throughout my life. Some of these issues are changing our World in an accelerated way, as we never thought it would happen. Metaphysics are no longer an "abstract theory with no basis in reality." Filmmakers and modern writers are exploring in-depth at one-time forbidden issues, and the gap between the real and 'could be' is shrinking.

The now accepted, scientific and popular of a Multiverse reality, or the existence of several universes, that some scientists affirm are in the thousands or even millions, is dramatically changing minds and opening up to real and speculative new dimensions or scopes.

We are, undoubtedly, living a revolutionary World, unfortunately, commanded by corrupt politics, full of greed, hatred, nescience, and irresponsibility. But, once again. I won't get into politics. They have already ruined a good part of our society.

That brings us into an inner study of our material body, and the marvelous connection with the spirit soul, thru Consciousness, being the brain the executor of the physical body functioning.

This wondrous link that many of us are only starting to discover and use it as an advanced tool for wellness is becoming more and more a reality to enjoy and make it work in our benefit.

It is a pleasure and privilege to me, to be able to write about it, so the people that already know

about it are getting confirmation of

its advantage, and the ones who didn't know about it could start to discover a new avenue to improve their lives, aging healthy and in style.

80's Are The New 50's

(If you prepare in advance)

CHAPTER 5

The eventualities.

Eventualities are the inevitable unannounced, mostly obstacles we encounter daily in our way.

They are practically unavoidable; Sometimes they are enjoyable, other times bring problems or concerns.

As I was writing a new chapter, I had to take care of some personal health issues. I was compelled to use my philosophical skills and some concepts I've been writing about in previous chapters.

A few weeks ago, I woke up with severe pain all over my body, but especially on my upper left back and chest, opposite to the rear main point of discomfort.

The general feeling suggested a feeling like a Semi-truck had run over my body. As I mentioned before, I usually take a very hotly morning shower, especially hitting my lower back for a few minutes. It helps my body with a 'tune-up' like effect.

So, that morning, I followed my usual routine. However, as the day progressed, the pain continued to bother me, this time with more severe intensity than average. I took a Diclofenac Sodium (or Voltaren) as I usually do on similar sporadically occasions. But the pain continued during the day and increasingly at night, preventing me from having a peaceful, relaxing night sleep. The following morning, the pain continued to be present, and I noticed that the focal point was changing places from front to back and sometimes even on the left side armpit.

The following day, the pain increased in intensity. In my mind, the origin was muscular, but just in case it wasn't, I emailed my Cardiologist describing the pain and asked her for a suggestion.

Dr. Kim suggested me to take some pain killer (Tylenol) and if the symptom continued, to go to the E.R. for an evaluation.

I took an Ibuprofen, since I didn't have Tylenol at hand, and the pain reduced in intensity. The next day, as I repeated the dose, I noticed some blood in the stool. That afternoon, I decided to check into the Emergency Room at Mount Sinai West.

After the initial Triage process, a doctor came, and I explained the situation to him.

Immediately, the doctor recommended a Cat-Scan. He said: "Here in the E.R., we got to make sure we find the 'bad stuff' first."

In a couple of hours, the results showed up, discarding any heart malfunction or other dangerous events.

However, none of the doctors could identify the cause of the pain.

Ready to go back home, and while they were processing the official release, I went to the bathroom and once again, my stool was sitting in a pool of blood. I showed it to the E.R. doctor. Immediately, he stopped the release papers. After a quick phone call, he came back and said: We're going to keep you here for the night. We will perform a Colonoscopy/Endoscopy in the morning.

Both tests were planned a couple of months before by my Cardiologist. However, because I am under blood thinners to prevent a possible stroke due to my Atrial Fibrillation condition, the first scheduled time for the exam failed. The anesthetist refused to do his job concerned by the blood thinner. A couple of days later, because I stopped the conflicting drug two days before and not three days as advised, again, at the last minute, they refused to conduct the procedure.

Whoever went to the preparation for this method, knows that the previous steps are the hard ones. One must ingest one gallon of liquid, no solid food or any non-transparent liquid for a whole day. It's not pretty, and you have to stay the day practically permanently sitting on the bowl. Then, upset by the incidents, I decided to postpone the Colonoscopy for a while. However, the related events at the E.R. decided my fate quickly.

So, the next morning, they took me to the procedure room, I was put to sleep, and I woke up two hours later. It seemed to me that nothing had happened. In a few minutes, the doctor came in and informed me that the procedure had been a success — no dangerous diagnosis.

However, still, no one knew the cause of my pain that persisted, once the effects of the anesthesia passed.

The whole event of my stay at the E.R. turned into an interesting experience. A learning lesson for an avid observer like me.

Looking at those patients coming to the E.R. Most of them looking in pretty bad condition, brought my attention to see that in most cases, the patients looked worn out. Principally like they were ready to quit; with no hopes and scary for their future.

The Emergency room, with all the expert doctors and technicians, and even the additional workers helping them on peripheral tasks, are prepared to save lives. The team works like a clock, with precise directions and fantastic coordination. It is almost miraculous how they act, virtually like triggered by a spring, executing their assignments automatically and without doubts.

We should praise the E.R. teams with high honors! They deserved them!

My observation of patients coming and going focused on something I have been writing, confirm my thoughts once more. The brain is the center of operations within the body and the Commander in Chief of our desire to stay healthy and enjoying this material life. Something that I didn't feel most of the E.R. patients strongly had present or visible.

I hope I am not wrongly judging patients I saw in the E.R. during my stay. Incidentally, the person I had next to me in the hospital room, before the procedure, was a very difficult one. His attitude was conflictive. He argued with the nurse and the doctor in rather rude terms, that watching the professionals dismay, made me believe the guy was unreasonable. Finally, in a rage, the patient took his I/V off, changed clothes, and suddenly left the hospital, without following the discharge rules.

The nurse and doctor looked at me in despair as they left the room. I didn't dare to ask what was the problem. I assume, by listening to part of the conversation, the patient was unreasonably demanding and wouldn't take any advice from the doctor and nurse.

People have the choice unless they refuse to think or unable to reason with clarity, to take the different ways to live a good quality life or not. However, due to Karma, those choices are limited or already decided. It's unfortunate, but also true.

Curiously, we are living a present time where especially youngster prefer to live an intense short life rather than a long existence. I can see why, however, it is not clear to me what the reasons are.

The U.S. Health System is hugely complicated, and ignorance of the rules make it even more challenging to understand it. I, myself never realized how the whole thing works.

Somehow, I have some clear understanding: If you don't ask, chances are, you won't get it. Never take no for an answer and keep asking for what you believe you deserve, within reason. Some times your demands won't be satisfied, but persistence is advisable. In only one week, the Mount Sinai system performed on me an array of procedures and tests hard to believe. A Cat/Scan, Endoscopy, Colonoscopy, MRI, Renal Ultrasound, various blood lab. Tests and a dermatology exam. And I still have scheduled a visit to a G.I. physician.

Wow! I am grateful to my doctors and the Mount Sinai System.

When the pain began, two weeks ago, I decided to stop writing the book. Because I thought: I can't continue to talk about my excellent condition until I learn the truth. At the same time, because the health care of one's body is so complicated, I decided that my readers would like to know the truth. Notably, the eventualities that can alter the ordinary course of life.

Despite the unexpected event, bringing a virus to my body that was causing severe pain, my brain kept sending the positive signals that called for a return to a healthy body. My previous writing was continually telling me that a defensive attitude was a must to get better soon.

Although the pain was excruciating, especially at night wearing out my energy, the use of pain killers was not the right option.

They would irritate my stomach provoking bleeding. Pain killers
only mask the pain but don't eliminate it.

I was hoping my new primary care physician, who I was scheduled to see for the first time in a few days, would help to solve my problem and stop the pain.

Three days later, I went to the Clinic for my first appointment with Dr. Heather Viola. She impressed me from the first moment of my visit when I asked what did she needed to know about me. Dr. Viola responded: well, I probably know more about you than you think. I read your clinical history, and I think I'm up to date. Then, she continued, I believe you have a viral infection in your stomach, and we are going to get rid of it. You will be taking some antibiotics for 14 days, and in the end, you will come to see me for a new evaluation. She gave me some hope.

She was able to pinpoint the problem; a stomach viral infection that reflected the pain to the already described places. I asked how was that she guessed the issue since the Endoscopy report only said: 'Stomach irritation.' Then, she said: Well, there is also some information in the biological inform.

She prescribed the necessary medicines, mainly antibiotics, which I am taking as I write. They almost destroyed my guts, but the infection seems to be gone.

I picked up the prescriptions from the Pharmacy and added those to the usual ones I take for my heart condition and Diabetes. I also take supplementary dietary food as Flax Seeds Oil and Cinnamon capsules to help Diabetes.

The fourteen days supply was a kind of torture to my stomach, and only my desire to get better kept me on track until the end of the series.

Those two weeks seemed to be endless. I read several times the previous chapters of this book, and I must confess it

helped me to keep the focus on my daily brain decisions.

Slowly, my body was positively reacting to the antibiotics, allowing me again, to have some nights of rest, and good sleep.

I diminished gym activity to compensate for the loss of energy caused by the massive dose of antibiotics, although they were helping me to manage the pain in my back and chest. Still, after the gym workout continued to be present.

I must confess I never felt this kind of pain, so steady and intense that was draining my energy even more than ever before.

The E.R. time had a significant impact on me, binging me to reality and the fragility of life and health.

That piece of amazingly complicated machine that is the human body, although it could be managed to a certain point by the brain, the final destination it is up to the individual Karma. Some call it destiny.

The Ancient Vedas say that we have a Karma. It is a complex mixture of past deeds and desires that at the very end of one's life, whatever is our honest hope or wish in our mind, will determine the outcome of our next existence and surely in what kind of body we will re-incarnate. Of course, nobody came back to tell the story, but when we have a choice, we must make a decision. That is why it is so important, being in a positive state of mind at all times.

During my short two days stay at the hospital, I had the chance to talk to many doctors, about my pain and also of general issues. Of course, some asked me about my activities, which I described thoroughly, especially about my writing activity. One of the physicians, Dr. Amita Buddhedev, an Academic Instructor at Mount Sinai, showed especial interest on the book I'm writing, mainly on the link between the brain as a Commander in Chief, as I define it. After talking for a few minutes about it, she encouraged me to continue the writing, saying that many patients at the hospital would be interested in knowing my ideas and asked me to let her know how she could get a copy of it after printing. I promised to deliver her the printed book personally.

Surprisingly, I am finding out that what initially, I thought that what it was a crazy, bland idea, little by little it was becoming an exciting theme for an entertaining and in a certain way, educational book for patients.

It is known, even on Highly Scientific circles, that we only use 10% of our brain capacity. It would be quite challenging to understand why, and also how scientists could affirm the truth of such evaluation. It is, nevertheless an old reputable opinion going around for many years.

Lately, because of the intense developing of spiritual concepts and philosophical schools, including the ancient Vedas re-discovery, happily recovered from under the dust of aged Libraries, we can retrieve this priceless information, disappeared for many generations.

The knowledge contained in this fantastic literature is helping humanity to keep up with sensible data and principles for life in this World and beyond.

Consciousness, a word that in most dictionaries appears as "the state of being awake and aware of one's surroundings."

"She failed to regain consciousness and died two days later" synonyms: awareness, wakefulness, alertness, responsiveness, the sentence "she failed to regain consciousness."

Or: the awareness or perception of something by a person, a superficial, simplistic description of its true definition, has a concealed meaning linked to the spiritual energy, that lately is gaining respect in Scientific Circles. The word is a description of the link between the spiritual, and material energy increasingly accepted to represent a forgotten concept that explains the spiritual power as the one that infuses aliveness in a body. We could resume the idea of the absence of life in any given dead body, to the lack of a soul, the invisible but present energy that differentiates the status of a mass of inert flesh and bones to the vigor of a moving, breathing body pumping blood and oxygen thru its vessels.

Fortunately, things are changing, especially with the humongous amount of information and knowledge carried by the Internet, helping to practically uncover dramatic details from the ancient Scriptures, buried for years in the darkest places on Earth.

In a very humble way and making absolutely no claim of personal credit, this writer finds pleasure to unveil the knowledge learned from the reading and studying of The Vedas. It is my sincere hope that it will help people to understand life better and have a happier life, destroying the standard popular belief that "ignorance makes people happier" a 'mirage' like, fashionable false statement. It takes a while to learn the benefits of education, but once you achieve knowledge, nothing compares to it.

So, finally, almost a month since the narrated episode began, I am gradually regaining my usual strength and going back to my regular schedule. I can feel it in my abdomen. It is starting to feel firm and therefore giving me the power that for a few weeks, I thought would never come back.
Nevertheless, consistent with my philosophy of turning any event, even the most negative one, into positivism, I am

saving the experience learned from the crisis and the confirmation that the brain is always the driver inside the body, of course, linked to the soul thru Consciousness.

Of course, training is a must.

But, you must look for the strength within your soul. It is there. Just search with faith and determination, and you will find it. Our creator planted it in our existence.

80's Are The New 50's

(If you prepare in advance)

CHAPTER 6

Listen to your doctors.

I'm happy to be back to my regular schedule, after the events narrated in Chapter 5!
I can't thank enough all the doctors involved in the episode. It was scary for a moment.
Following their directions and the collective actions was an experience that I would like my readers to treasure and

learning from the new style of Medicine Practice.

It has been a long road from the days when I grew up when one General Practice doctor had to know most areas and intricacies of medicine and specialists were just a few, taking care of very critical tasks. Nowadays, things are very different and the way they work, as teams of doctors, each one focused on targeted sectors of the body that amplifies the scope and deepens into the particular problems encountered. The teamwork, of course, is limiting somehow the general personal activity, although it increases the opportunities for success in diagnosis and treatment by physicians consulting and feeding back each other with information and opinions. As I wrote before, the work observed in the E.R. is an excellent example of medical teamwork.

Providing your doctors with accurate information about how you feel, where your problems seem to be located, the pain degree, or any indication that will help the physician to identify the issue, and would be the best way to help them to know how to detect, localize and to treat the problem. Consider that your feedback and information to the Physicians are most essential for them to learn what is affecting your body, and help you to cure it. Nevertheless, the patient is, ultimately, in most cases, the one that will carry the responsibility to overcome the illness. It also includes some elements impossible to control, like certain diseases or actions of Karma.

Always remember that the brain being in control helps to keep an orderly action and positive attitude, undoubtedly helpful to a prompt recovery.

A proper exercising schedule is also an essential part of keeping the body young and healthy, and following a smart routine, is a fundamental part of it. There will be some times when you don't feel like exercising, however, then is when you must force your brain to impart the right directions to drag yourself to the gym, or a walk in the park rather than hang-out and skip the workout. Once you are at it and start moving, your body will follow the usual cycle effortlessly. Most problems could be solved by a walk thru Central Park or any park.

Don't let laziness to make the wrong decisions. That's why I emphasize that the brain is the commander in chief. Nevertheless, it is a retrofitting action where Consciousness decides which way to go.

I am sorry if I'm complicating things a bit, but I find it difficult to express my mind in a more precise way. It is not an easy subject.

All I wish to transmit to the readers is that taking the right decision at every step of the way is a combination of body and mind, being the brain the engine, powered by the soul, thru Consciousness. It reads easily to me. I hope it also does for you.

Hygiene is a critical part of the whole process. It is what maintains a sanitary

condition and promotes order in your home and workplace. There is no possible success unless you keep a neat and orderly place around you. Also, a good personal appearance is an encouragement to continue with the desired assignment. I don't mean an obsessive, vane daily personal grooming. But, if you look good to yourself, you will also look good to others, and open up for success.
It is not a matter of vanity. It is a convenient habit.

Sexual activity is also a vital part of life, even as you age.
Of course, when you get older, chances are you might lose your partner or spouse, and at a certain age becomes challenging to find another suitable companion.
An old friend used to say: "You have to solve your sexual problems the best you can." I leave it up to each one of you to decide the interpretation of my friend's words.
However, the body has its philosophy and expresses the daily needs, which in the case of sexual activity, there is a natural

decrease as the body ages. However, libido never goes away.

Sigmund Freud established that libido is a part of the person's id. To Freud, it represents all psychic energy and not just sexual energy.

But, in modern days, this energy can be controlled and managed by the brain, choosing the right moves that after going thru the period of life where the individual's id, is obeying natural laws of species' preservation and reproduction. My education is Liberal/Conservative, meaning that although I observe Conservatism, I am also open to new concepts, which I study, taking some and discarding others. I believe the primary purpose of sex is procreation. However, our creator has made sexual relationships immensely attractive, almost impossible to refuse, and the trigger to eventual copulation; to preserve and defend the species.

Common sense and other personal and
social factors are deterrents or selectors of
the possible consummation of a sex act.
Nevertheless, age is another factor
determining the course of events.
Besides the fact that after a certain life
period, children are not desired, for
apparent reasons, sexual intercourse
becomes an exclusive pleasuring act, and
therefore an optional choice. Sexually
transmitted diseases are also deterrents,
especially for people that are not fans of
condoms or having troubles using them. I
am one of them. Therefore, many of us
have chosen to stay away from sexual
intercourse, dedicating our intellect to
other activities that at a certain age are
more fruitful and rewarding. Also, hoping
we will encounter our rare soul-mate to
share a late experience. Still, for some
people, at one point, self-gratification is
another option upon incidental cases.

Another subject to consider is cosmetic
surgery. It is widely known that altering
what the Creator has given us at birth is
sacred and we must religiously take care of

it; many people are falling in the trap of trying to keep looking younger and improving their appearance. Although in rare cases this type of surgery seems to work temporarily, although, after a few years, the consequences of the procedures are undoubtedly showing inevitable disgraceful looks, sometimes scary and an evident proof that there is nothing better than what nature has given to us at birth. That also goes for the so-called Transgender, a condition that in my humble opinion is nothing more than a fantasy; an attempt to live in an imaginary world, that although people have the natural right to adopt, it doesn't go beyond imagination, and feelings.

Also, the surgeries and hormone treatments that the mentioned individuals go thru, trying to change the unchangeable, have terrible consequences, many times lethal.

Those artificial hormones, exceptionally wrongly given to children, are a crime to human beings unable to choose their destinies and becoming objects of foul play by their insensible, parents, irresponsibly trying to fulfill their own frustrated personal fantasies, forcing children to transit dangerous ways. How can a person chose gender sides when they don't even understand what sex is for?

As my readers had the opportunity to evaluate my thoughts and experiences up to now, some of you might like them; some may not. From the beginning, my intention is to give a realistic view of my life choices, that have worked for me, and it could work for some of you.
Life options have changed radically in the 20th century and keep an accelerated transformation as we go thru Century 21. Some may like it; some might not. However, there is nothing we can change, or do about it, and the only option available is to accept it as it is, trying to adjust our personalities, tastes, and results, making personal decisions that will help us to get the best out of this imperfect world we are living.

For the ones that believe in life after death, we surely have an advantage. If we are right on our belief, we are living a better experience, thinking that our souls will not evaporate. For the ones that don't believe in life after death, well, that will be it, folks. No additional time. Game over!

One more thing! As I went thru these pages, over and over, proofreading, correcting, adjusting and expanding, I had the opportunity to follow my suggestions and counseling, finding comforting to take advantage of my recommendations to my readers.

For instance:
One of the subjects referred to in earlier chapters that have helped me to improve my health in the stomach virus incident is the use of natural antibiotics like Turmeric, Ginger root, and Cardamon. A combination of those three potent powders enabled me to finish the treatment of the stomach viral infection that Dr. Viola

108

initially stopped with chemically known prescription antibiotics.

The first dose, taken for 14 days, got rid of the gross infection. However, something like a shadow of the pain remained in my system, always present, and although the pain was only a fraction of the primary stages of the problem, depending on the position, I could still feel it in my back. However, my system was saturated with the powerful antibiotic's prescriptions, so, I decided to try my own recommendation in an earlier chapter.

As soon as I finish the prescribed 14 days dose, I began taking a coffee spoon of the three herbs powder mentioned, diluted in orange juice, first thing in the morning. Little by little, the pain shadow diminished substantially. One more proof that natural antibiotics work as an aid to potent prescription drugs. It is essential to understand that herb therapy is not a substitute for medicines prescribed by doctors. However, they have proved to be a useful complementary aid to our health.

I believe this book is, overall, a sincere narration of life experiences, that I hope will be useful and enjoyable reading.
If you find the experience helpful, please don't hesitate to express your feedback. It would be highly appreciated, even if it is not great.
See "Important message to readers:" on page 11.

Thank you for staying with me thru the journey narrated in this book.   I hope you enjoyed the ride, as much as I did writing it!

J. Pelegrin

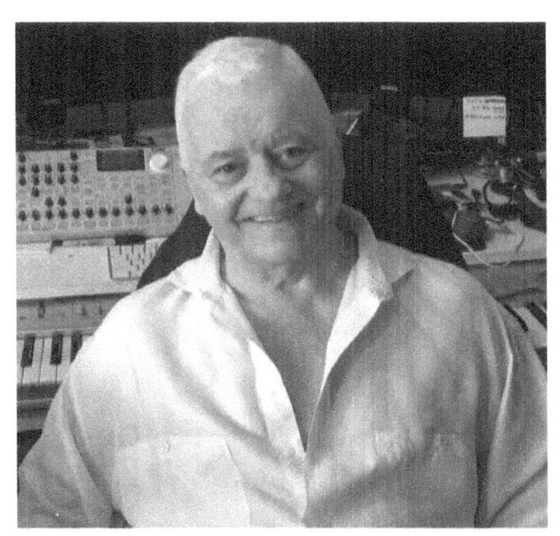

ABOUT THE AUTHOR

J. Pelegrin creative history goes back to the beginning of the group "LOS 4 BRILLANTES", formed in Uruguay in the 60's: Yvonne <Lead Singer> Roberto <bass>, Ricardo <guitar> and me, Jorge <keyboards>. Then, a little later we added Hector (drums), who accompanied the Group and later was an integral part of it until the end, by 1970's.

They began playing and singing in Uruguay, their homeland, traveling to Argentina, Brazil, Chile, Venezuela, Perú and landing in Mexico, in 1964, where they remained until 1970 when decided to go separate ways.

CBS Columbia Records Mexico hired Jorge as a Producer-Artistic Director. After two years, working for the label, having produced several successful projects, encouraged by his Boss, he decided to move to New York, where he founded a successful new home. Jorge's relationship with New York City was "love at first sight." Since 1974 to the present has been his home, except for eight years, between 1989 and 1998, were he had to take some time off to attend to family matters, back in Uruguay.

New York City has been a great deal in Jorge's life. It brought him the opportunity to develop himself into a better musician, a writer, and a better person, giving him the recognition

and success in the English Language
market, that to these days had helped him
to complete many of his dreams,
including writing Newspaper articles,
books, and making movies. He is very
grateful to New York City and its people.
In New York, he had the fortune to have
produced five hit records for the
American Market and some others in the
hit parade top 40's: "WALKING
DOWNTOWN," featuring "Black Ivory,"
"IF YOU WANT ME," by "Ecstasy,
Passion & Pain." "FEEL GOOD, PARTY
TIME", by J.R.Funk & the love machine."
"ROCK YOUR WORLD", by "Weeks &
Co" and ""I DON'T WANNA LOSE IT",
featuring "Wayne Cooper", former late
"CAMEO" lead singer.
In 1998, returning to his beloved City of
New York, destiny took him thru various
ways until he came back to his heart and
soul: the music. In 2005, with best friend
Sue Samuels, a dancer, choreographer and
multi-talented NYC icon, they approached
something new. They began to write a;
Broadway-bound Musical Play, (THE
DREAM FACTORY).

By 2008, they finished the writing and composing the music and lyrics. Some Broadway producers read the script and listen to the music of the play and immediately showed interest in producing the show. They offered to assign an expert budget director and Executive Producer, thinking on a production budget of 5 million dollars and the request to do it fast since they needed to replace their fading Broadway play: "SPRING AWAKENING," after seven years on stage.

Unfortunately, 14 days later, the Real Estate "Market Crash" surfaced. Jorge and Sue received a notice saying that due to the World's economic situation, the project had been postponed indefinitely (All the investors were people affected by the Wall Street collapse). The market crash shattered their dreams.

Affected by this disappointing fact, Jorge began a life reorganization, which besides the Musical Play setback, that leads Jorge to his personal life collapse, ended in a bankruptcy and three consecutive brain strokes.

Changes in the entertainment market took him to other new ways, were taking advantage of the Electronic Music escalation, he began to produce Music Videos, Film production and, combining his music creativity, the writing and the new visual aspect of it.

He released his first Music-Video production on Youtube by April of 2012. Being that the Music business is in frank decadence, the music production has fallen to an unrecognizable mediocrity. A few productions in today's market have a decent quality and the rappers, managed by obscure characters who own most record labels or managed to

merge with unscrupulous big Media Corporations CEO's, have monopolized the pop music market, it became irrelevant to keep producing music for the American Market as a way of living.

Instead, the book industry has begun to pick-up, and Jorge now dedicates his time to the book writing. He has written a

Musical Film Script, with 23 original songs, titled: DREAM FACTORY, selected by the 2015 Beverly Hills Film Festival, as the best Musical. Then,
he wrote a political/Religious book: "SAVING AMERICA THE BEAUTIFUL, a Fiction Novel: "DEATH IS ONLY AN ILLUSION", and "Postmodern LIBERALISM" published on Amazon Books.

AMERICA GENIAL! POR SIEMPRE
Versión en Español de
KEEPING AMERICA GREAT!
"URUGUAY PUERTO LIBRE" in Spanish Language, an essay on local Uruguayan economy.
"DREAM FACTORY", a Musical Film Script, Selected as the best Musical at the *2015 BEVERLY HILLS FILM FESTIVAL.* Include 23 original songs.
"SAVING AMERICA THE BEAUTIFUL", a "current affairs" narrative about Jorge's arrival to New York City, the process of integrating to the community, his progressive interest in politics, and the Donald Trump stomping the grounds in the political arena. J. Pelegrin predicted the election's result on July 4th, 2016.
"Postmodern LIBERALISM" (An Obsessive Epidemic)
Postmodern LIBERALISM" (An Obsessive Epidemic)
"DEATH IS ONLY AN ILLUSION", A Fiction Novel.

Synopsis 1

When Martin Frost, a Philosophy professor at an NYC University closes his class and lecture year, in a speech to his students, he quotes "DEATH IS ONLY AN ILLUSION," from the Vedic philosophy. Some curious students want to know more about the subject and invite the Professor to expand on the theme privately. A visitor from an alternative Planet appears on the scene, looking for help to stop an imminent invasion by Earthlings' Terrorists to take over his Planet.

The Alien invites Martin and friends to visit his Parallel World; the group enjoys what they see and commits to helping. Some student's parents, former CIA operatives, join the Professor and friends to form a "Garrison" to aid the man from the Parallel Planet to defend his remote homeland. Exciting action, high in Philosophy, Sciences, Religion, Morals and unexpected developments in an electrifying thrilling plot.

ALSO AVAILABLE: - TAMBIÉN DISPONIBLE:

"LA MUERTE ES SÓLO UNA ILUSIÓN"
"DEATH IS ONLY AN ILLUSION's", en Español

www.ingramcontent.com/pod-product-compliance
Lightning Source LLC
Chambersburg PA
CBHW031130250726
48655CB00002B/600